DAM THAT HABIT

HOW TO MENTALLY REVERSE
THE HABIT OF SMOKING CIGARETTES

BY

RUDWAAN

Author: Rudwaan
Publisher: Move The Village
Website: www.thelionstale.com

Edit and Format: Rodney Piggott

Manuscript prep: Rodney Piggott

Cover Design: He Ruler
getseenandheard.com

ISBN: 978-0-9900279-3-5

CONTENTS

Chapter   **Page**

DAM

DAM THAT HABIT

HABIT

This Book Is For You

You may know of someone who feels trapped in the grip of indulging the urge to smoke cigarettes. The Pharmaceutical Industrial Complex, the Medical Industrial Complex, the Tobacco Industrial Complex and the Governments of so-called developed countries like the U.S.A., China, Japan, England are all in bed together on steering yourself, your loved ones or your friends down the path of medication as a first response to ending this grip.

Not only are they all making a fortune on the consumption of cigarettes, they have devised a way to make a fortune on your futile attempts to quit when you use their prescribed medicated methods such as the gums, patches, and e-cigs.

This book introduces a monkey-wrench into this scheme when the steps are applied and adhered to, it shares with the reader three simple psychological steps to take that will cause the mind to **reverse** the urge to smoke cigarettes, and this is done without the use of drugs and has a permanent effect, with no negative side effects.

I wrote this book to help others escape the illusion that they are addicted to nicotine. This is the lie that keeps the mind from even trying to rid itself of an unwanted habit.

Once you believe that you cannot change your condition without the use of drugs your mind shuts down any attempts to do otherwise, and this is chi-ching $$ for those collaborators who conspire to keep you in the dark. This book sheds light on some truths that will set you free, if you have the will to be free.

Have you tried to quit smoking cigarettes only to fail time and time again? Were there times when you thought this is it, because a month, three months, nine months, several years went by with no cigarettes? Not that you didn't feel the urge from time to time, but you stuck to your guns, you showed that cigarette who was the boss of you.

Then one day, perhaps your stress load was excessive, you lost a valued job, you caught your spouse with your best friend, a loved one transpired, something brought the urge to smoke back into your conscious mind as if it was always there, you picked up a cigarette and puffed away without the need to re-learn how to smoke, you did not experience the feelings you had when you smoked your very first cigarette as a teenager, you did not choke, you did not feel like passing out, in fact you felt as if for the past three months, nine months, or even years you had not actually quit smoking, it's as if the habit had not gone anywhere, it was still in your mind waiting for the perfect opportunity to re-engage the urge to smoke, **it was in fact like riding a bike.**

If you can identify with the above sentiment on some level, then this book is for you. This book is for those who really want to rid their lives and the lives of their love ones of the detestable and deadly habit of smoking cigarettes, for truth be told when you smoke cigarettes so too do the ones you love and virtually everyone you come in contact with thru 2nd hand and 3rd hand smoke, we will explore what these are in coming chapters.

This book is for those who have tried all of the 'this arrest' and 'that arrest' medications, you've tried the patches, the gums, the hypnosis, you may have even called the psychic network, you've tried and tried and nothing produced that permanent effect of cessation.

If you suspected that you may have been addicted to nicotine, these failures have now convinced you that you are hopelessly addicted to nicotine and the only way out is to submit to one of the ever emerging medications for the remainder of your life and suffer the side effects, after all Big Pharma will have the drug to manage the side effects of the drugs you took to manage the side effects of the drugs you took to help you quit, whew! If you are ready for a way out without all those side effects, then **this book is for you.**

I encourage you to read this book in its entirety, not just once but multiple times. **The wordings have been carefully selected to open your eyes to truths that have been deliberately hidden from you**, simple truths that once unveiled will elicit 'aha' moments. Moments of such intense clarification that your mind will begin to organize itself to promote them to you like billboards on the highways and backroads where the urge to smoke travels to your consciousness. The language is very simple so that one does not need a psychology degree to understand what is written. The mind tends to reduce input to absolutes and absolutes are often simple, uncomplicated.

 Here are what you may expect reading this book will do for you:

- **Reading this book will empower you**. Information is power, and this book will give you information grouped in such a way that it has no choice but to make sense to your mind.

  Imagine walking along a path and finding a half of a dollar bill, then three months later along the same path you find the other half of that same dollar bill, your mind may not prompt you to associate the two and form a whole dollar, in fact you may have forgotten and may have discarded the half of the dollar bill you found three months ago.

Now imagine again that walking along the same path you find a half of a dollar bill, you already know where I am going, that's the simplicity that is so empowering, then five steps later you find the other half to that same dollar bill, your mind will more likely promote to you that the two halves may be associated, so you will follow your mind's promotion and match the two to see if they form a perfect match, and when they do you will have an 'aha' moment.

The 'aha' moment is when you consciously acknowledge that your mind's promotion made sense. We assign different terms to this moment, we may say things like 'I had a gut feeling' or 'I felt the urge to…'

Much of the information in this book you may have heard or read somewhere at some time, but because the information was not presented in steps, and may have been accessed months or years apart, your mind did not prompt you to form an association of the bigger picture, each time you encountered such information was like the first time to your mind.

You will find empowerment within these pages not only due to the information presented but due to the inherent association between the pieces of information presented, this is why I urge you read and re-read to draw out the 'aha' moments. Those 'aha' moments are moments of empowerment.

- **Reading this book will help you to determine how you got where you are.** The error made by many attempting to 'get rid' of the habit is that they don't know 'where they are' and 'how they got there', so Big Pharma and its collaborators make an insane fortune by promoting to you that you are where you are not, because you don't know how you got where you are you don't know how to re-trace your steps, so the same entities that benefitted immensely from getting you where you are, they are the same ones giving you the steps to get you to another place where they can take more of your money.

  Because you don't know why you have such an intense urge to smoke cigarettes, the chances of you smoking again after simply quitting are likely. Reading this book will help you to answer the crucial questions for yourself, this book is not designed to simply give you the answers, it presents information in such close proximity that your mind will naturally form the association and it is this formation your mind makes that is crucial to reversing the habit.

- **Reading this book will help you find your way back.** Reading this book will help you determine how you started to smoke cigarettes so that your mind can see how to not just quit, but reverse it. Reading this book will help you determine where you are in regards to smoking cigarettes, are you 'addicted' or do you have a 'habit', knowing where you are will enable your mind to take the best route out. Knowing why you acquired smoking cigarettes will enable and empower you to never go that way again, therefore this method has a permanent outcome with no side effects.

- **Reading this book will help you to help yourself.** This is most important to grasp, most if not all physiological methods devoted to smoking cessation such as the 'patches' and 'gums' promote to you that the help you need is outside of yourself.

  They tell you that you will never do it without their help, they assume power over you and because they have not assisted you in answering the crucial questions of 'how, where, and why' you willingly submit your will to their destined-to-fail methods and assume a spectator role waiting for them to fix your problem.

  Reading this book will help you see that a great part of why you are where you are can be directly attributed to a subdued will. By applying those destined-to-fail physiological methods that simply make more money for Big Pharma and its collaborators, you are simply trading one harmful subjugation of your will for another.

  Applying yourself to the information and suggestions within this book puts you and your mind in the driver's seat, fact is, you and your mind drove you to your current destination, and it is you and your mind armed with the empowering information within this book that will drive you out of it, isn't that empowering in and of itself?

Finally let me tell you briefly **what this book will not do for you.**

- **This book will not lie to you** and tell that the information within is some great 'secret'. The steps I will share with you are simple and easy to apply yourself to, the only requirement is that you be ready to rid yourself and the lives of your family, friends and co-workers of the detestable habit of smoking cigarettes.

- **This book will not re-direct the power away from you.** This is not a program to upload to your mind, or some invasive technique controlled by an outside manipulator. You will not be hypnotized and given post-hypnotic suggestions that can have a damaging effect on sleep and eating patterns, no one but you will have power over you.

- **This book will not set you on an impossible course of action.** You will not be at odds with your mind, the steps in this book will not direct you to fight your own mind. Many programs and techniques direct you to 'trick' your mind, to 'suppress' your mind, they put you at odds with your mind. This book will remind you that your mind never wanted you to engage in this habit in the first place, your number one ally in your struggle to free yourself from this detestable habit is your mind, you don't want to fight it, you want to do just the opposite, you are on a mission to rescue your mind from the illusion it is trapped in. **This book will show you the way**.

My Story

Once upon a time I smoked cigarettes. My story is much like yours. As a young boy growing into young adulthood, I crossed path with others who smoked cigarettes, I remembered riding the bus dreading the smell of the smoke, in those days it was permissible to smoke cigarettes on public transportation, the smoke was noxious, smelt awful and caused me to choke, and this was just 2nd hand smoke.

The smoke would burn my eyes. I could not envision myself ever smoking one of those awful smelling cigarettes. Some of the people I observed smoking looked sickly, they coughed frequently, and some had really bad teeth and awful smelling breaths. Some of them had blackened lips and spoke with a coarse voice. I would later learn that these were your **die-hard smokers**, they smoked so much and so often they could not smell the stench of their own breaths.

I soon encountered the recreational smokers, these were classmates and church-mates, they seemed normal enough, no incessant cough, no stained teeth, some even dressed better than I did. I was at that vulnerable age in my life, the point of trying to fit in, trying to be cool, to be down with the 'in-crowd' as much as possible yet stay off the parental-radar.

Some of the teens from the church I attended smoked cigarettes recreationally, they kept the chewing gums and breath sprays to mask the scent, and some would even have a bottle of sample cologne in their pockets to further mask the cigarette smoke from their parents.

The peer pressure was very subtle, no one forced me or dared me to smoke. Sneaking out of choir rehearsal, or ducking out of a service to go 'light one up' was almost like a sport in and of itself. I had to get on the team so I tried it, yes, just like you I choked, I thought I was going to pass out, or throw up, 'how could anyone think this was cool?' what was that cold feeling? Why was everyone else just inhaling and exhaling as naturally as breathing fresh air? I had to master this sport to get on the team, to earn my 'cool' points.

So I tried it over and over again, my peers were only too eager to allow me to 'bum' from them over and over again, they would coach me on how to inhale. Finally, I could actually make it thru an entire cigarette without feeling cold all over, where did that cold feeling go? I could smoke an entire cigarette without choking. I didn't even notice the habit setting in, it was so subtle, but soon enough mastering the smoking of cigarettes would be the least of my worries, I was now buying my own pack.

I wrote this book because I've been where most of you are. After seven years of smoking cigarettes I tried quitting over and over again. The longest period of cessation was eight months, I thought I had it beat that time, but one day I bummed a cigarette and was back at it as if I never stopped, no cold feeling, no choking, **it was like riding a bike.**

After that final time trying to quit, I decided to go about things differently, I was always fascinated by how the mind works, this fascination led me to structure a course of action that began to yield surprising results, not only was my daily ration decreasing, I was also feeling very good, enlightened, it's as if I could finally see the light at the end of a very dark tunnel.

What I had actually done without setting out to do so was reverse the habit, I literally found myself back on the other side of the habit, the side where I found the smoke reprehensible, all those feelings I had about cigarettes before I smoked them were still there, the feelings of disgust and repulsion. The big difference is that I was no longer at that vulnerable age where peer pressure could influence me to do something I initially could not see myself doing.

I started smoking cigarettes at the age of sixteen, I reversed the habit at the age of twenty-three, I am now over fifty and I have never felt the urge to smoke a cigarette after the reversal and I know that I never will. The reversal is a permanent effect with no side effects.

I defined the steps I took and introduced them to a few friends who were also ready to rid themselves of cigarette smoking, the results were the same, permanent reversal of the habit with no side effects.

With the high cost of cigarettes, the decline in socially acceptable places to smoke, the increase in awareness of the debilitating effects of smoking, the time could not be more perfect to introduce these proven steps to help those who are ready to rid themselves of the detestable habit of smoking cigarettes.

This book will help you to define yourself. Most of you think as I once did that you are addicted to nicotine. This book will help you see that what you are is habituated to the urge to smoke cigarettes, this is a very powerful and important distinction. Once you gain clarity on your position as I did, you will see where you came from, and with a little help from this book, how to get back home.

Up in Smoke

Here are some reported facts about cigarette smoking that is important for your mind to associate together. You may have heard or read most of this information, but when grouped together the information tends to have a lasting effect on the mind. The truth is that every day countless lives are literally **going up in smoke**.

- Cigarette smoking may kill close to **1 billion people** in the 21st century if current trends continue '*source*: *International smoking facts*' **an insane amount of money will be made by the Tobacco Industrial Complex and its after-market while those 1 billion people are slowly on their way to their graves.**

- More than $9billion *usd* spent on advertising and promotion of cigarettes annually. Young teens are the primary focus of the Ad campaigns. '*source: FTC*' **is there a conspiracy to get teens hooked on cigarettes to replace the adults who are dying every day from cigarette related diseases?**

- Each day over 100,000 young people start smoking cigarettes as a daily habit, these are young people who have gone beyond the initial stage of trying it out, **so each month over 3,000,000 teens start the daily habit of smoking cigarettes.** '*source: World Health Organization*'

- Smoking cigarettes can lead to disease, disability, and death, it can harm every organ of the body. '*source: USDHHS*' **This is guaranteed income for**

Big Pharma and the Medical Industrial Complex.

- As many as 7 in 10 adult smokers want to stop smoking cigarettes *'source: USDHHS'* **After making a fortune from your smoking habit the collaborators are primed to make an additional fortune from your destined-to-fail attempts at quitting. They get you coming and going.**

- More than 600,000 non-smokers die each year from 2nd hand smoke worldwide. *'source: ASH'* **Fact is you are killing not just yourself but your loved ones, your friends, your co-workers, the innocent bystander you don't even know.**

- There are about 7,000 toxic chemicals in cigarette smoke, let's just name a few: *'source: World Ed.'*
  - **carbon monoxide** (car exhaust)
  - **tar** (makes roads)
  - **arsenic** (rat poison)
  - **ammonia** (cleaning products)
  - **hydrogen cyanide** (gas chamber poison)
  - **cyanide**
  - **acetone** (nail polish remover)
  - **butane** (lighter fluid)
  - **DDT** (insecticide)
  - **formaldehyde** (embalm fluid)
  - **sulfuric acid** (car battery)
  - **lead**

- Tobacco Industry revenue can average about $74billion *usd* annually *'source: ASH'* **with any industry there is an aftermarket that makes a fortune, for example the auto-industry after-market does not make cars, but they rely on the**

car-manufacturers to make their money, you will need a battery, windshield wipers, tires, car-wash etc. In the same way Big Pharma and the Medical Industrial Complex do not manufacture cigarettes, but they make a fortune from cigarettes being manufactured and consumed. So why would they want to help you get off the hook?

Now that you have given a small fortune to the Tobacco industry and are ready to give up smoking, Big Pharma and the Medical Industrial Complex ride in on their smoky white horse and present you with some options. Your doctor may recommend any of the existing medications to help you manage your 'nicotine addiction' that does not exist. **This is the 'smoke and mirrors', as long as you are convinced that you are addicted to nicotine your only hope is to try one of these medications**. In trying to avoid death by cigarette you invariably put your life on the line when you submit to one or more of the popular medications.

Here are a few of those choices and their related side effects:

- **Chantix:** This is a smoking cessation drug made by Pfizer. Some common side effects are; seizures, insomnia, **suicidal thoughts**, nausea, unsettling dreams.

- **Nicorette:** Made by GlaxoSmithKline. Some common side effects are; irregular heartbeats, nausea, weakness, mouth sores, sore throat, hair loss.

- **E-Cigarettes:** An unregulated product so anyone can put one of these on the market. This is a liquid nicotine-like substance in a toxic chemical cocktail, 1 tbsp. can kill an adult, there is no quality control, causes lung damage, contains some of the same harmful toxic chemicals as cigarettes, contains toxic metal Nano-particles from the vaporizing mechanism.

These are just some of the popular options you will be steered towards as you embark on the quest to rid your life of the detestable habit of smoking cigarettes. Not only is smoking cigarettes big business, but your attempt to quit is also big business.

So much so that the Tobacco Industry is openly vested in the manufacturing and promotion of E-Cigs, what other smoking cessation aids are they invested in? Don't think for a minute that they are concerned about public health, not when they are still vehemently opposed to stringent regulation.

Their goal is simply to make lots of money, and they will make money from your smoking habit, and they will make money from your attempts to quit. I want you to see the smoke and mirrors, if they are playing these games with your very life what else could they be possibly lying about?

Why would you expect the industry and its after-market to truthfully identify to you why your attempts to quit end in destined failure? Continue reading, I assure you that the truth will set you free.

Nicotine: The Fall Guy

Nicotine is the 'fall guy' for the Tobacco Industry and its after-market, they dare not tell you who the real bad guys are, **because if they did smoking cigarettes would be as popular as sucking on your car's tail-pipe.**

Let's put this fact right up front, there are many popular foods that contain nicotine, you read that right, some of those foods are; tomatoes, eggplant, cauliflowers, potatoes, and most other foods from the night-shade family. The same nicotine found in tobacco is the same nicotine found in tomatoes, so ask yourself 'why aren't you addicted to eating tomatoes?'

Is the nicotine in tomatoes a kinder gentler version of nicotine? is it a vegan form of nicotine? The answer is a resounding no, it's the same nicotine found in tobacco, the difference is you don't add 7,000+ toxic chemicals such as formaldehyde and ammonia to your tomatoes then smoke it.

Nicotine also has many medical benefits, it is used for ulcerative colitis, depression, schizophrenia, pain, mild cognitive impairment, Alzheimer, and Parkinson's disease.

This gives you a different picture of this dreadful and deadly cancer causing nicotine you are supposedly hopelessly addicted to.

You've seen the movies where that one unsuspecting guy is left holding the bag, he doesn't benefit from the crime, but he is the one who gets caught and does the time. The real bad guys are not mentioned on the 6 o'clock news, instead they get away with all the money and are sunning on some exotic beach, this is what they are doing to nicotine.

Cigarette smoke contains over 7,000 deadly toxic chemicals that have no other use but to kill, but the 'fall guy' is nicotine, the same nicotine found in tomatoes and potatoes and has medicinal benefits, that's the only chemical that causes cancer and addicts you, according to those counting the money, arsenic and butylene to name a few have nothing to do with your cancer, really?

The truth is if nicotine was such a bad guy then tomatoes and cauliflower should come with warning labels from the Surgeon General, the public should be warned that eating tomatoes may lead to cancer, but you will never see such a warning label on tomatoes and the other foods that contain nicotine because nicotine does not cause cancer no more than drinking water causes cancer, if, however the water contained over 7,000 chemicals such as arsenic and cyanide then drinking that water may cause cancer.

Let's peel back the proverbial onion a bit further while we are on the subject of 'fall guys', just as the tomatoes would not be the bad guy after being laced with 7,000+ toxic cancer causing chemicals, so too **the real tobacco** is not at fault either. To the native peoples of meso-America tobacco was considered a 'gift from the Creator'. The tobacco smoke was seen as carrying one's thoughts and prayers to the Great Spirit.

Besides spiritual applications tobacco was used in ethno-botany, for medicinal treatment of physical conditions, used as a pain-killer for ear-aches and tooth-aches, used as a poultice, used for treating asthma and tuberculosis. Tobacco was also used as currency.

The commercial value of tobacco came with the arrival of the Europeans, with commercial use came competition, with competition came branding, with branding came chemical additives to flavor and alter the natural chemical structure of the plant. The tobacco used to make cigarettes is a hybrid that no longer functions as the original naturally occurring tobacco.

The commercialized 'curing' process of this plant produced 'Advanced Glycation End products' (AGE) which contributes to atherosclerosis and cancer, wow! cancer comes into the picture way before nicotine is even a factor, the potential for cancer is identified in the commercialized methods used in the cultivation of the tobacco plant that will be used to produce cigarettes, the potential for cancer comes in way before the 7,000+ toxic cancer causing chemicals are added when manufacturing the cigarettes. Is nicotine really the bad guy or the fall guy?

The commercialized cultivation of tobacco adds to the potential of cancer and other diseases to the smoker. The chemical fertilizers used to enrich the soil for faster growth **(there's money to be made who has time to wait on mother nature)**, insecticides used to kill pests, artificial flavorings used to distinguish brands, and don't forget the chemicals used to keep the tobacco burning as a cigarette.

No wonder when a large commercialized tobacco farm stops producing tobacco the government mandates that no other food item can be grown on that farm for 50 years due to the sheer amount of harmful chemicals in the soil. After growing and harvesting the hybrid tobacco with all those chemicals they then add 7,000+ toxic chemicals to produce cigarettes, but they want you to believe the smoke in the mirror that nicotine is the bad guy.

But now you know the truth, keep reading, you are well on your way to freeing your mind from the urge to smoke cigarettes.

The Smoking Gun

Your will-power is growing as you continue to read this book, information presented in an associative way is empowering to the mind. Let us continue along this path as we climb higher up the mountain and go deeper into the rabbit hole. We will now drive a wedge between two terms that have been deliberately interchanged to confuse and shroud your mind in an illusion so that drugs that have physiological effects can be marketed to you to solve a psychological problem.

- **What is a habit?**

  Habit is defined as *'a constant often unconscious inclination to perform some act'*. This act whether it is good or bad is acquired thru its frequent repetition. The key word in this definition is *inclination.* Inclination is *'an attitude or disposition towards something, having or expressing mental tendency'*.

In the above paragraph 'habit' is clearly defined for us courtesy of Webster's dictionary. Nowhere in the above definition do we see such phrases as 'uncontrollable desires' or 'impossible to control urges', instead we see 'inclination'. Whenever you are inclined to perform some act there is also a part of your mind that declines to do it, this is the law of opposites.

Picture yourself at the cross-roads, you choose the road you take, the road does not choose you, the road does not force you to choose it, you make a conscious choice. If you choose to incline yourself towards one road often enough the inclination to choose that road may become habitual, it may become comfortable to you because your mind will eventually form a comfort zone around that inclination, it may become as familiar to you as where you live.

After living in the same place for 5 years how often do you find yourself trying to remember where you live? There is a direct correlation between the term 'habit' and 'habitat', this is not a coincidence.

The habit, good or bad, once acquired is like a home to your mind. The power I'm revealing to you here is that choosing to smoke cigarettes consistently or your inclination towards smoking the cigarette becomes the habit, not necessarily the act of smoking the cigarettes itself. This is why no matter how many cigarettes you smoke daily, you may be a chain-smoker who lights up every 30 minutes, but when you go to bed at night you sleep thru the night without waking up every 30 minutes to smoke.

The smoker who is in the hospital hooked up to machines with their legs strapped up does not tear themselves loose just to go have a cigarette, what happened? The fact is the mind is not trapped by the act but by the inclination or urge to commit the act, in so doing when the mind senses that the body is not in a position to engage in the act the mind temporarily suspends the urge until such time as the body is in the position to engage the urge.

It is very important and empowering that we understand how a habit is formed before we can successfully reverse it.

A habit whether it is good or bad is formed simply by the frequency with which you incline yourself to perform the act. Therefore, the act itself is not as relevant as the inclination towards the act. Your mind has formed a comfort zone and has made itself at home (habitat) around the inclination, the urge, **it is this inclination that has your mind trapped, not nicotine**.

When you are through reading, fully absorbing, and applying the steps in this book, you will be fully empowered to manipulate the habit of smoking cigarettes for your own good. **Habit is formed due to a degree of psychological dependency. In other words, it is the mind that is trapped.**

- ## What is addiction?

    Per Webster's dictionary the word addiction stems from the Greek word *addictus,* when we break this word down to its components we will have an in-depth understanding of what it means to be addicted, we can then compare addiction to habit and drive that wedge between them so you can see where you actually are. If you are convinced that you are addicted when in fact you simply have a habit, you are apt to seek the wrong treatment which may then lead to further physiological complications.

Let us look at the first part of the word '*add*' Webster's defines this word as *'to join or to unite so as to increase in size, quantity, or scope'*. The second part of the word is '*ictus*' Webster defines this as *'a sudden attack, a fit, or a stroke'*. This is a pathological term which simply indicates that the body or brain is directly involved, unlike **habit** in which the mind is directly involved.

Let me take this time to briefly but adamantly state that it is not my intention to diagnose, prescribe, or treat addictions, the traditional definition is merely being explored in an effort to form a comparison with habit and thus highlight the wedge that exists between these two conditions. That being said let us look closer at addiction.

Unlike habit, addiction can be instantaneous depending on a variety of factors such as dosage, strength of the foreign substance, and or chemical make-up of the individual, these are just some of the factors that may play a part in the time it takes for addiction to a substance to establish itself.

Under addiction the brain's natural behavior is altered, even if the mind is dead set against performing the act the brain will evoke a strong enough **'ictus'** that demands the individual **'add'** more of the controlling substance to the brain's satisfaction, we will explore why this happens.

This is how it works; the brain does not recognize the foreign substance that is being ingested, if that substance is of sufficient potency or other factors described above are present, the brain begins to spend an inordinate amount of time trying to figure out what to do with what is being ingested.

The brain may even begin to abandon other duties to the body in order to have more brain power devoted to figuring out what to do with the foreign substance. When the level of the controlling substance drops below a benchmark set by the brain, the brain evokes an **'ictus'** which is a fit or a stroke literally forcing the individual to **'add'** more of the foreign substance to the brain's desire before the 'ictus' will be appeased. If not for this 'ictus' most people who are addicted may be able to walk away, the 'ictus' is characterized as 'withdrawal symptoms'.

The brain may manipulate this benchmark by raising the bar requiring more 'adds' and more frequently. The brain becomes trapped in a vicious cycle of what I term the **'pseudo supply and demand cycle'**.

There is no intention here to take the severe and complicated state of addiction and reduce it to a simplistic view, I am simply exploring the word itself as it is used in connection and comparison to the word habit. Your empowerment towards freeing your mind from the trap it is in depends a great deal on you being able to distinguish addiction from habit.

The Tobacco industry and its after-market driven by Big Pharma are hedging that you do not know the difference between these two conditions, and so they are able to market drugs to you that affect the brain when it is your mind that is trapped by the urge to smoke cigarettes. If you do not successfully see the difference between these two terms your ability to successfully reverse the habit may be hampered, simply because you will apply the rudimentary definition of addiction to the term habit. In short you will continue to label your habit as an addiction. **Addiction is established due to a degree of physiological dependency.**

In our exploration of habit, we noted that habit is formed due to **a degree of psychological dependency**. Simply stated, the mind is trapped by the inclination to commit the act.

Furthermore, from our observations it is quite evident that to a degree **the act itself is not as potent as the inclination**

or urge to commit the act, this is why in certain cases when someone attempts to 'cold-turkey quit' the habit they may pick-up another oral fixation such as sucking on tooth-picks, chewing gum, or excessive eating.

Since the urge is still there the mind simply attaches it to another oral expression in order to continue feeding the urge, that person in most cases may go right back to smoking cigarettes.

As part of my research I conducted several interviews. One woman I interviewed had 'cold-turkey quit' smoking for 15 years. One particular excessively stressful day, she was on her way home driving by the same store she would buy cigarettes from when she did smoke, she stopped her car, went into the store, bought a pack of the brand she used to smoke, opened it up, and lit up.

She said it was as if she was having an 'out-of-body' experience, as she watched herself go thru the same ritual she would engage in 15 years prior to that moment.

I helped her understand, as I hope you will, that quitting is easy, in fact every night you go to sleep you quit smoking, you do not, I hope, wake up every hour or a couple of hours just to have a cigarette, now if you were addicted, and that addiction was as strong as the Tobacco Industry and its after-market would have you believe, you would be up all hours of the night maintaining the same schedule of smoking as during your waking hours.

Since it is not the act of smoking but the urge to smoke that the mind is hooked on, the mind merely suspends that urge whenever you are not in a position to engage the urge. That means if you chain-smoke during the day, when you go to sleep the urge to smoke will be put on a high shelf until you wake. If you are in the hospital hooked up and bed-ridden, your mind will suspend the urge to smoke, you will not experience such violent 'ictus' because you are not addicted, you have a habit.

So every night when you are asleep the urge to smoke is temporarily suspended, for those 6-8 hours you 'quit' smoking.

When you 'put your foot down' and insist that you will no longer engage in the act, your mind knows that to front burner the urge when you have 'made up your mind' not to smoke will simply produce undue stress, your mind is not your enemy, it knows you are the boss of it, one of your mind's jobs is to make you comfortable, so your mind will simply put the urge on a very high shelf, higher than the nightly shelf it uses to turn off the urge while you sleep or are otherwise unable to engage the urge, but the urge will still be there, that woman's urge was on a high shelf for 15 years.

Some trauma, or something very subtle such as a memory, can shake that urge down from that high shelf at any time, be it a month, eight months, or 15 years, the urge can be re-engaged, and when it is, it is re-enforced, now Big Pharma and the Medical Industrial Complex can really peddle the 'addicted to nicotine' lie to you, you may never try to rid your life of this detestable habit again.

There are some circumstances that can cause the mind to put that urge on such a high shelf it might as well not be there, but it is. It will take a quake that moves the entire planet to bring that urge down.

One of my interviewees was a Great-grandmother who chained smoke, she would smoke any and everywhere, she would smoke around the children with no regard, she had to have that cigarette, after all she was convinced she was addicted to nicotine.

One day her Great grand-daughter who was about 4 years of age at the time was playing dress-up, she had on a big hat that swallowed her head, was wrapped in a shawl, and was attempting to walk in Great grandma's shoes, she said 'grandma look at me', when the Great grandmother looked at her she could not help but laugh until she saw what her 4 year-old great grand-baby was holding in her hand, between her fingers away from herself just as she did, her little precious Great grand baby girl was holding one of her cigarettes, putting it to her lips mimicking smoking the way she did.

Her heart almost stopped, in that moment she realized what her smoking behavior was leading to, her 4-year-old great granddaughter was going down the same detestable road she was trapped on, in that moment she grabbed all of her cigarettes, broke them all up and flushed them, when I interviewed her she had not smoked a cigarette and did not feel the urge to smoke in about 5 years. She was 87 at that time and may very well transition before any such trauma of sufficient potency moves the urge, that is still there, down from that very high shelf in her mind.

The point here is that quitting is not the problem, because the mind is not as concerned about the act of smoking as it is about the urge to smoke. This is why you hear so many stories, and yours may be one of them, as mine was, of people attempting to quit only to return to the habit after a few months or a few years, these attempts actually re-enforce the notion that one is addicted to nicotine.

Fortunately, the information shared in this book will enable you to escape this illusion of smoke and mirrors.

There are good habits, such as exercising, eating foods beneficial to the body, going to bed at a reasonable hour etc, and of course there are bad habits such as cigarette smoking, staying up late watching Tv, eating foods not beneficial to the body, some people have a habit of 'cussing' **a habit good or bad is established due to a degree of psychological dependency**, the mind forms a comfort zone around the urge to perform the act. This is a very crucial and empowering piece of truth, the mind does not form a comfort zone around the act, but around the urge or inclination to commit the act.

There are only bad addictions, there no good addictions. Under addiction the brain functions as an enemy of the body, **addiction is established due to a degree of physiological dependency.**

Under addiction performing the act is most relevant, the brain must have sufficient amount and dosage of the controlling foreign substance to appease the 'ictus'. Ones state of mind is irrelevant under addiction, though the individual may have 'inclined' themselves initially, once the brain is hooked the inclination is no longer a factor.

In some cases, such as crack cocaine, the individual may have inclined themselves once, but due to combined factors such as the potency and perhaps their chemical make-up, the brain was instantly hooked. There are other unfortunate circumstances, such as babies born addicted, where the person's inclination never weighed in. Once addiction sets in it is the brain that must be weaned out of the trap I call the 'pseudo supply and demand' trap.

A great percentage of smokers are average to recreational smokers, a lesser percentage of smoker's chain smoke several packs a day, many of them succumb to death or serious impairment from the over 7,000+ poisonous chemicals they have been sucking into their lungs day and night for 20+ years, the nicotine did not kill them, the arsenic, cyanide, formaldehyde and other poisonous toxic chemicals found in cigarettes killed them.

A Smoking Hand

At the card tables of Vegas, a 'smoking hand' is most desirable, but with the cigarette smoking habit **2nd hand and 3rd hand smoke are deadly to those around you whether they smoke or not.** Let's briefly examine how your smoking habit really and truly affects those around you and why.

What is 1st hand smoke?

This is you smoking your cigarette drawing the smoke thru the filter, some of the poisons are trapped by the filter so the smoke entering your lungs is not as potent as the smoke coming from the unfiltered tip and consuming the oxygen in the air.

Notice how you hold the cigarette away from your body, away from your face, because if the smoke from the unfiltered tip enters your lungs undiluted you too will choke, so you protect yourself by holding the burning tip away from yourself.

You know there is nothing truly tasty about cigarette smoke, you do not try to gulp the smoke in the air, you do not put the unfiltered tip to your nose and mouth and try to suck it in because it is so good, no, you suck the smoke thru the filtered tip and hold the unfiltered tip where the full force of the noxious smoke is away from your nose, ask yourself if you the smoker can't stand the smoke coming off the unfiltered tip how then can that child or your co-worker? **1st hand smoke is the cigarette smoker drawing the smoke thru the filtered tip while those around them are exposed to the smoke from the unfiltered tip.**

What is 2ⁿᵈ hand smoke?

This is the smoke that everyone around the smoker is exposed to, this includes the smoke they blow into the air, and the smoke coming off the unfiltered end of the burning cigarette. **Studies show that each year over 660,000 persons die from 2ⁿᵈ hand cigarette smoke.** The most dangerous 2ⁿᵈ hand smoke is the burning unfiltered tip, because at the burning unfiltered tip the poisons are not being filtered, so 100% of the noxious cocktail is spilling into the air and into the lungs of those breathing the same air as the smoker.

The smoker who is ready to rid their lives of this detestable habit must use this fact to help them, do not ignore it, allow your mind to associate the information shared in this book, you are a good person engaged in a very bad habit that may not only kill you but may also kill others around you, your smoking habit may very well be the cause of someone else developing lung cancer, brain cancer, or dying, your smoking habit may impair the growth and normal development of a child, perhaps your child. **2ⁿᵈ hand smoke is the 1ˢᵗ hand smoker involving mostly innocent bystanders, who depend on the same air for life, into the dance with death that they are engaged in.**

What is 3ʳᵈ hand smoke?

This is a relatively new area of study that I did not know existed when doing my research. I actually unveiled it by research and labeled it 3ʳᵈ hand smoke only to find out that someone else also thought of it.

3ʳᵈ hand smoke is the smell of the cigarette smoke that lingers long after the cigarette is extinguished. It's the smoky smell in your hair, in your clothes, in the car, in your room or house. When we smell something we are actually taking in molecules of that thing thru our noses which warms the air and turns those molecules into a liquid which then enters our olfactory system, forms 'odorant patterns' which are then sent to the brain.

According to **Medical Daily** '*Smell is regarded as one of the most powerful and evocative senses; it can behave as a time machine of sorts in triggering memories, and aids in attraction, love, and sex. Its inner workings are considered more complicated than that of an airplane*'.

Consider that little child you constantly pick-up and hold close to your smokey smelling hair and or clothes, that child smells the cigarette molecules which are warmed in their tiny nostrils and turned to liquid form for travel to their still forming brain, consider that you just gave your little baby girl or boy, your grandson or grand-daughter a small but still deadly dose of the noxious cocktail containing over 7,000+ toxic chemicals which includes the likes of lead.

Consider also that smell forms emotions and may function as a time-machine where feelings are evoked of perhaps pleasant memories when the scent is present. Let's say you are your grand-child's favorite person, they love jumping in your arms, but every time they do you have that certain smell, the smell of a noxious deadly cocktail of chemicals that to them is like a sweet smell because it reminds them of you, do you see that you may be planting the seeds of smoking cigarettes in their mind that may be triggered to remind them of you at some point in their lives? **3rd hand smoke is the 1st hand smoker inadvertently dosing those who get really close to them with a mild but still deadly** cocktail of the noxious and toxic smoke from the cigarettes they smoke.

3rd hand smoke can also be delivered by those who are around cigarette smoke enough so that it settles in their hair and clothes, but who do not necessarily smoke themselves. The cocktail waitress or bartender for example.

Smoke Signals

During my research I identified at least 5 types of smokers, though they all respond to the urge to smoke the urge itself is largely triggered by a particular atmosphere. While the smoker may experience several mini-triggers to engage the urge the atmosphere must be right to begin with otherwise those mini-triggers will not activate the urge. These types I label as follows:

- **The Casual Smoker,** this is the person who may smoke a couple of cigarettes a day, maybe no more than 4 or 5. They will say they smoke just because they want to, they enjoy a good cigarette every now and again, they will say that they can quit whenever they want to, that they do not really have a habit, smoking to them is just another thing to do occasionally, like chewing gum.

  If you tell this person that smoking cigarettes can kill them they will tell you that you can get killed by crossing the street. The 'Casual Smoker' and the 'Recreational Smoker' below account for about 80% of smokers in most societies.

- **The Recreational Smoker,** this is the person who smokes only in fun environments such as parties, backyard barbecues etc., this person does not smoke at work, nor at home, and what is of utmost importance is that the urge to smoke does not present itself in any other atmosphere other than a fun-filled atmosphere.

This person may not even buy cigarettes because they go stale for lack of smoking, so this person is the proverbial 'bum' at parties and fun-filled atmosphere who will 'bum' a cigarette from the person they are standing next to who is smoking.

- **The Nervous Smoker,** this person only smokes when they are feeling nervous like before a test or speaking engagement. This person is convinced that in order to calm their nerves they need to smoke. What they fail to realize is that with each pull of those noxious chemicals it brings them that much closer to heart failure, their blood pressure actually increases as the noxious smoke saps the life-giving oxygen in their blood, that's the cold feeling of death that their mind hides from them in order to support the comfort zone it has built around the urge to smoke.

  The urge to smoke is triggered when this person feels nervous about something, at first it may have been crucial things such as a big test or presentation, then the slippery slope sets in and they are nervous for no obvious reason or for things they weren't always nervous about. This person's excuse for smoking is that they have 'bad nerves'. The 'Nervous Smoker' accounts for about 5% of smokers in most societies.

- **The Time-Waster.** This is the smoker who does not fit the background of the average smoker, they may not have begun smoking as teenagers and now they are full grown adults, so while the average adult who never smoked may never smoke, this adult picks up the habit because they are in an environment where they cannot just pick up, pack up, and leave whenever they want to.

This may be the person who finds themselves incarcerated, or serving in the armed forces. Because those environments are so confining and smoking cigarettes is the thing to do to dissipate time, this adult who has never smoked may find themselves responding to the subtle cues to smoke.

The mind forms the comfort zone around the urge to smoke just the same. One of my research interviewees was a gentleman who did not smoke when he came home on leave from active duty, but when he returned to the confines of the environment the urge to smoke greeted him, and he engaged it. The 'Nervous Smoker' above the 'Time-Waster' and the 'Specific Situation Smoker' below may all account for about 10% of smokers in most societies.

- **The Specific Situation Smoker.** Not the same as the time-waster or the recreational smoker, the urge to smoke only presents itself when the individual is in a specific situation.

I formed this category around an interviewee who only smoked when he attended his family re-union, though he has been a guest more than once at other people's family reunions the urge to smoke did not present itself there, only when he attended his family reunion once a year did the urge to smoke appear.

So this was a person who only smoked once a year, and when he was there at his family reunion he would smoke as if he had been smoking all year, no choking or feeling dizzy, it's as if his lungs were fully acclimated to the noxious smoke, this is how powerful the mind is, once it forms a comfort zone around the behavior, thus establishing the habit, it will mask the negative feelings from you.

- **The Chain Smoker.** Lastly, this is the smoker whose mind is firing the urge at them contiguously, every cigarette is like the first cigarette for the day. The important take away from this is that this is still a habit, we are still dealing with the urge to smoke, a mental dependency, we know this because this person still goes to bed and gets at least 6-8 hours of sleep, so while they may smoke every 30 minutes during their waking hours they do not wake up every 30 minutes to light up.

If the cause of their chain-smoking was this 'addiction to nicotine' that the tobacco industry and its aftermarket wants us to believe then the brain would be trapped and when the brain is trapped it relies on the chemical to be at a threshold in the bloodstream otherwise it will trigger 'ictus' after 'ictus' until the person 'adds' more of the controlling chemical to the brain's satisfaction. The habit has reached a critical level with this type of smoker and may very well lead to death or severe impairment.

The 'Chain Smoker' may account for 5% of smokers in most societies, there are societies in which smoking cigarettes is as commonplace as drinking water, those societies will not conform to this percentage breakdown.

No matter the category you identify with you are still dealing with a habit, in some, the habit may be more or less intense than in others. Even though the mind is in a trap it is still protective, so the teen who has the urge to smoke when they are around their friends at school or otherwise away from home may not feel the urge to smoke at home or any place where their parents may be present. This is why there are so many categories, I have presented the major ones most smokers fall into, those categories themselves may also have sub-categories.

Let us now go full speed ahead into the techniques introduced to you to help you 'reverse the urge' to smoke cigarettes. I will be introducing some new terms that you have never heard of before, these terms are used to pull the habit apart into its component parts, then using, not fighting against, the power of your own mind you will surely see the habit fall apart, lose its grip on your mind and then blow away like dry leaves in the wind.

Now that we have sufficiently fed your mind enough pertinent information that when grouped together and viewed at one time, instead of months or years apart, provides powerful tools to draw upon as we step into the main course where I will guide you thru three simple but powerful steps. I labeled these steps 'mental dams' and these dams will naturally and without force cause your mind to reverse the urge to smoke cigarettes.

The results will be that once again the 'see-saw' will have your will to 'decline' to smoke heavily outweighing your will to 'incline' to smoke until there is no longer a see-saw to contend with, just as you were when you could not even imagine yourself ever smoking those nasty, smelly cigarettes.

The major difference now is that no amount of outside influence can pressure you into smoking cigarettes no more than you can be pressured into sucking on your car's exhaust.

Smoke Trails

We are now entering the application phase; it is very important that you do not skip any steps presented in this work.

Our first step is visualization, it is very essential to your success that you visualize your beginning, most average smokers share a common beginning, most started as teenagers when their minds were susceptible to peer-pressure, the average person did not come bouncing out of the womb with cigarettes on their mind.

Most smokers had a strong disdain for cigarette smoke, most everyone can remember choking when others smoked around them. No one walked into a smoky room and sucked in the air and said 'ah! What a lovely smell' Who enjoyed smelling the breath of a smoker? I'm sure you didn't either, these are the memories I want you to conjure up, they are still in your mind because that is the original state your mind was in before you insistently and consistently inclined it towards the urge to smoke.

Go back to your very first cigarette, do you remember the process? It's similar for almost everyone who smokes. Let me help you remember how you got where you are; you were young, probably a teenager, you struggled with the decision to try it, a small part of your mind was inclined, a very large part of your mind declined to try it.

Picture yourself on a see-saw, your inclination to smoke was outweighed by your declination to smoke, your mind knew that this was not a good decision, it was like playing Russian roulette, who says 'gimme that gun?' Your inclination to smoke was dangling in the air on that see-saw like a light-weight child, not heavy enough to influence your mind, after all you always felt that cigarette smoking was disgusting.

The smoke from the cigarettes of others caused you to gag, the smoke smelt really foul, probably because a lot of feces is found in the tobacco used to make cigarettes. If you remember other negative feelings you had towards cigarettes before you acquired the habit it is useful to bring them to the forefront of your mind at this time, envisioning your mindstate before your mind got trapped by the urge is very useful towards freeing your mind of that trap.

Focus on the fact that with all of the negative feelings you had towards cigarettes your mind would not have been inclined towards performing the act, your mind's declination outweighed the small inclination that your vulnerable young impressionable peer-pressure susceptible self was exposed to.

Did you need help with that first pull? That help may have come from peer-pressure, or teenage issues such as school-work, perhaps you saw your parents smoke, some outside pressure encouraged or emboldened you to take that first pull, whatever the source, one thing was for certain, your mind's declination towards not smoking was temporarily outweighed.

I say temporarily because that one time did not form the habit, the see-saw was only temporarily moved in favor of the inclination, once the outside pressure was no longer around the see-saw would swing back in favor of your mind's declination, the inclination would once again return to dangling in the air like a small child.

In reality your mind's declination to smoke is still heavier than its inclination to smoke at this juncture, I need you to visualize your story along these lines.

Now take a moment to fully absorb and digest what I have just shared with you, we have journeyed back to your beginning, the more visual you are able to conjure up that time of your life the more effective this journey towards freeing your mind will be. Do not go beyond this chapter until you fully understand it, and are able to vividly see where you came from, how would you know where to go back to if you can't identify where you came from? This is what is so empowering about this book, it is you who are in the driver's seat of your mind, as it should be.

My purpose thus far has been to clearly reveal to you what a habit really is, to take you back to your beginning of your cigarette smoking habit, and help you visualize yourself crossing over for the first time, by this time you should have experienced one or more 'aha' moments, one such moment should be that the first time you inclined yourself to smoke did not establish the habit of smoking.

It was vitally important to take you back to the beginning because it is from this memory that you will find the power to reverse your steps.

From the beginning you will see that your mind's position was over-ridden, **because you can consciously override your mind's position,** and thru frequent, consistent and contiguous over-ridings it adapts and forms a comfort zone, the habit, around the inclination.

It is empowering for you to know that your mind always wants you to feel comfortable, operative word is feel, whether you are actually comfortable or not is irrelevant, as long as you feel comfortable the mind does not perceive any stress from the activity, that doesn't mean the stress is not there.

Within the comfort zone the mind will not front burner the negative effects of the behavior to the conscious aware you, it literally hides the truth from you, because you (the boss) insisted on inclining to do what the mind (your servant) was dead set against in the beginning.

This is why recalling the beginning is so important, remember the dizzy feeling, the nausea, the cold feeling caused by the smoke consuming the oxygen in your blood, where did that all go? Your mind is protecting you from the stress of the truth, the first time you smoked was so traumatic to your heart and your brain as they were denied the amount of oxygen they needed to function. That reality still exists after years of smoking, cigarettes are even more toxic today.

You brought yourself that much closer to death with each pull on that cigarette, any of the over 7,000+ poisonous toxic chemicals can cause you to have a major stroke or heart failure with every pull on a cigarette, your mind allowed you to feel every uncomfortable stressful feeling in hopes of dissuading you from trying it again. Please believe that every time you smoke death still fingers your heart and brain, your mind just shields you from it within the comfort zone it formed due to you insisting.

By now it should dawn on you like 'aha', that a habit is mentally oriented, therefore it must be controlled, enhanced, or reversed mentally. Now you know why all of the other physical applications such as patches and gums are doomed to fail from the onset, the only thing they do is make a lot of money for the Tobacco industry and its after-market Big Pharma.

The Situational Habit

The actual act of smoking a cigarette is the **Major Situational Habit**, thinking about a cigarette, sucking on a toothpick or your thumb will not adequately satisfy the urge that the mind is trapped around, only engaging in the actual act is strong enough to satisfy the urge your mind is trapped around.

This is why I have labeled the act of smoking the cigarettes as the Major Situational Habit, this is the mother habit, and this mother habit or Major Situational Habit feeds the **mother urge**, which is the urge to incline to smoke the cigarette. Every habit is undergirded by the urge to incline that habit; the urge is likened unto the current under the wave. Read and re-read this part until you digest it.

The Major Situational Habit or the actual act of smoking the cigarette is not what your mind is trapped by, your mind is trapped by the urge to incline you to engage in the Major Situational Habit which is smoking a cigarette, picture your visualization of your beginning, remember the see-saw in which **'inclination' (do it)** was outweighed by **'declination' (don't do it)**, but due to you (the boss) consistently inclining, your mind eventually formed a comfort zone around 'inclining', this is the urge, which is like the current that runs under the wave, the act is the wave itself, but the current can move the wave to shore or away from the shore, it is the same current.

This Major Situational Habit could have been smoking or eating grass dipped in cow piss, the mind would have formed a comfort zone around your frequent, consistent, and insistent 'inclining' to smoke cow-piss grass. Your mind doesn't really care what the behavior is that you insisted on inclining, it builds a comfort zone around the urge.

This Major Situational Habit is supported and kept re-enforced by two Minor Situational Habits for most smokers.

The first is buying cigarettes, most often by the pack, the chain smoker usually buys cigarettes by the cartons. This Minor Situational Habit does not often pertain to the 'Recreational or party smoker' who often supports the Major Situational Habit by the second Minor Situational Habit of 'bumming'. Unless you make your own cigarettes you acquire the cigarette to smoke by either buying it or bumming it.

The reason quitting 'cold-turkey' and other methods hardly work is because the smoker attempts to get rid of the Major Situational Habit by going after the Major Situational Habit, the mind is trapped by the urge, the current under the Major Situational Habit, it has built a comfort zone around the urge to not just engage in the Major Situational Habit but also to protect it, it actually thinks it is protecting your interests since you are the one that insisted and persisted in the behavior in the beginning (picture your visualization exercise of the see-saw).

In order to reverse the mother urge (the current) to engage in the Major Situational Habit (smoking a cigarette) we must successfully reverse each of the minor urges to engage in each of the Minor Situational Habits in a specific order, then once those Minor Situational Habits have been swept out of the mind by the reversal of each underlying minor urges, the Major Situational Habit and its urge will subsequently be reduced to the strength of a Minor Situational Habit and its urge, then zapped like a pesky fly on the window sill of your mind.

Depending on the strength of the psychological dependency that the mind is trapped in, the mind will identify mini-situations or excuses that can be used to maintain the urge to engage in the Minor Situational Habit of buying or bumming which in turn maintains the Major Situational Habit of smoking the cigarette, for example after eating or drinking, before going to bed, sitting down to a phone call, taking a break at work, someone else lights up even though you just got thru smoking.

These are all mini-situations (not to be confused with the Minor Situational Habit) that the mind has identified as non-threatening to you, where you can safely and without negative external backlash engage in the urge to buy or bum cigarettes.

For example, such a mini-situation for some may be after or during attending church, inside the church itself is not identified as a safe zone to engage for most unless it's an office, not even the chain-smoker who feels compelled to respond to the urge every fifteen minutes will pull out a cigarette in the middle of the church and light up, but once outside of the church, while still on the church-grounds, perhaps a certain location has been identified as a safety zone that smoker will either take out a cigarette from a pack they had bought, walk to the corner store to buy cigarettes, or bum a cigarette so that the Major Situational Habit to smoke can be engaged in.

Do you see how that works? Read it as many times as it takes to wrap your mind around the process and see, perhaps for the first time, where you are, how you got there, then you will clearly see why the steps I will introduce to you on how to get back to the other side of the tracks is such a no-brainer.

The bottom-line is, in order to smoke a cigarette, you must have a cigarette to smoke. You will get this cigarette by either buying it or bumming it, if the urge is very strong then you may keep a fresh pack on your person so that you may engage the habit of smoking at will. If the urge is very weak you may simply rely on bumming or even buying 'loosies' which still falls under buying.

So we have successfully identified and introduced some crucial and powerful terms to you, we have identified and introduced the Major Situational Habit as the actual act of smoking the cigarette, this is the act that the urge to incline has wrapped itself around, in this relationship the urge is more important than the act itself, the urge can be and is manipulated by the mind to the comfort of the person.

This is why quitting is so easy and never permanent, because the mind can manipulate the urge, it does so every night you go to bed, you don't jump up every couple of hours to light up, the mind temporarily suspends the urge, it puts the urge on a high shelf so that you can get your required rest, but once you wake the urge is brought down from that shelf and it's back to smoking.

What happens to the urge of the smoker who has been in an accident and is hospitalized and bed-ridden for perhaps weeks? The mind knows that they are not in a position to engage in the act, not just because they are in the hospital, but because they have tubes running in and out of them. The mind knows that presenting the urge under these conditions when the person cannot possibly engage will only cause undue stress, and since one of the mind's mandate is stress avoidance it will shelf the urge temporarily, until the person is in the position to engage.

The same thing happens when the person says 'I quit' perhaps as a New Year's resolution, the mind senses that the person is very serious and will not cause undue stress by constantly presenting the urge, so after repeatedly refusing to engage the urge, the mind will simply put the urge on a very high shelf, this can last from weeks to months and even years, but the urge is still there, then one day the urge is triggered and almost trance-like the person re-engages the urge and begins smoking as if they never stopped, the comfort zone around the taste is still there.

Quitting is only a temporary cessation of the urge, what I will share with you is one if not the only permanent reversal of the urge known.

Here I will outline to you the steps we will take with the goal being to bring your mind to each crossroad, we know that one of the crucial roles of your mind is to make you feel comfortable, it does so by interpreting situations in such a way that the outcome favors you, without some strong outside force, like the peer pressure experienced in your beginning, your mind will always choose the path of least resistance, the path that is less stressful.

We will construct what I have labeled as **'mental dams'** at each crossroad that will cause your mind to choose the only accessible path which is the direction we want to go in. This process I have labeled **'mental steering'**, it doesn't matter that your mind knows ahead of time that this is what you are doing, once you continue to repeat the behavior that constructs the mental dam your mind will respond according to its mandate.

This is what the steps look like in short:

- Identify the Minor Situational Habit to be zapped
- Repeat the given behavior associated with constructing the mental dam as long as it takes
- The mental dam is constructed thru the repetition of the behavior and the natural outcome it produces
- The mind is at the crossroads and will make the only non-stressful choice which is to respond to the results of the behavior 'the mental dam'
- The behavior is directly associated with the particular Minor Situational Habit; the mind cannot end the behavior but it can end the urge undergirding that Minor Situational Habit which in turn ends the behavior
- The second Minor Situational Habit will automatically replace the first Minor Situational Habit because the Major Situational Habit still is in place
- We repeat the steps using the associated behavior
- During these steps we are also using a strict but flexible rationing system, flexible because we don't want the mind to become defensive, I also suggest flushing the lungs with exercise, plenty of water and fresh fruits, and using specific 'mind-awakening' language

- Once the final Minor Situational habit is zapped the Major Situational Habit by this time has been reduced to the status of a Minor Situational habit
- I introduce the final 'mental dam' that causes the mind to reverse the urge to engage in the act of smoking permanently.

Let's get started.

Mental Dam #1

Objective: To construct a mental dam that influences the mind to come to the conclusion that buying cigarettes is equal to throwing your money away literally.

You've probably already experienced others telling you that smoking cigarettes is wasting your money, it's like setting your money on fire. Your mind is prepared to deal with this rhetoric because the experience of 'setting your money on fire' is subject to interpretation, your mind tells you that drinking alcohol, buying candy, going to the movies etc are all wasting money.

There is a vast difference between someone telling you that you can die from lung cancer and actually being diagnosed with lung cancer and given a couple of months to live, one is rhetorical and can be dismissed the other is actual and the mind must and will deal with the reality. Keep this argument in mind when I introduce the actual behavior that will construct the first mental dam.

Preparation: The first thing you must do is determine your daily ration, remember you are not trying to quit, and you are not fighting your mind, your ration should be no more than roughly half of what you usually smoke on a regular day, do not determine your ration by an unusually stressful day in which you may smoke well over your usual amount.

This is the very first step you must take, do not go beyond this point until you have determined your daily ration, if you usually smoke ten cigarettes then your beginning ration may be between 5-7, this is just a suggested amount, if you feel you can begin with a lower amount then do so, but once you have started you may make no more than two adjustments to your daily ration that increases the amount you smoke. Do not choose a ration that is so close to your daily amount that your daily amount is practically your ration.

If you usually smoke an entire pack a day, where there is an average of 20 cigarettes in a pack then your ration should be at least between 10-15. It is very helpful to keep a log of your daily ration; this will be very helpful when you go over your ration or go under your ration. I will reveal why this is important when we go into the actual method. Set a start date and stick to it. Let your start date coincide with a day you need to buy a pack of cigarettes; you'll see why below.

Method: When your start date arrives go ahead and buy a pack of cigarettes as you usually do, count and keep your ration in the pack, crush, crumble, and render irretrievable, utterly destroy the excess cigarettes, yes you read that right, discard the excess cigarettes in a manner that renders them irretrievable, this may include flushing, soaking with bleach etc. Do not simply crush them and throw them in the trash because in your hour of need you will go back and find one in the trash that is smokable, they must be irretrievable.

Your mind will not fight this but your conscious aware self will object, you can only stop this behavior if you decide to give up, your mind cannot make you give up. At this time your mind is an observer of your behavior just like a friend may be, your friends and family may tell you that only a fool throws their money away like that, and that is exactly the conclusion your mind will eventually come to as you persist with the behavior.

Now I must warn you here, this will not work if money has no value to you, meaning, **if you are comfortable with taking a five, ten, or twenty-dollar bill and setting it on fire every day just for fun then this method is not for you**. This method is for those who work hard for their money, they have bills to pay, food to buy, maybe a family to support, they cannot afford to just throw money away.

But this is exactly what you do when you buy a pack of cigarettes, you get no nutrients from cigarettes, you ingest over 7,000+ harsh toxic chemicals like arsenic, you run the risk of developing lung cancer or some other form of cancer due to the toxic chemicals you are ingesting, you jeopardize the health and well-being of your family and friends around you, there is nothing beneficial about smoking cigarettes, therefore buying cigarettes is literally wasting your money.

Keep in mind that the decision to buy a pack of cigarettes is not a decision your mind makes for you, it's a decision you make, you can just as well bum what you need daily, the only thing your mind controls and is controlled by at this point is the urge to incline you to smoke, how you acquire the actual cigarette is up to you, your mind does not give one iota if you invest in a cigarette making machine and make your own cigarettes, it doesn't care if you work for a cigarette manufacturer and get them for free, so only the conscious aware you can decide to pull the plug on this method, I urge you to stick to it.

To engage the mind, the behavior must be consistently repeated, you cannot skip a day or two then start again, the mind will reset the clock if you do, when you successfully bring your mind to the crossroads where the behavior has constructed the mental dam, the mind is faced with a decision, to keep buying cigarettes is to keep literally, not rhetorically, but literally throwing your hard earned money away, every time you flush those cigarettes your mind will see $$$ going down the toilet.

The repetition of this behavior is what moves the mind to the construction site, your mind knows that there is only one direction to go in and that is to stop throwing your hard earned money away, remember, I stated that your mind cannot stop you from buying the cigarettes and throwing the excess away, but what it can and will do is reverse the urge underlying this Minor Situational Habit, remember, even though it is minor it is still a habit and all habits have their own underlying current or urge, your mind will literally reverse this urge from inclining to buy to declining to buy.

Remember, our overall goal is to influence the mind to reverse the direction of the Mother urge to smoke from 'incline' to 'decline' just as it was in the beginning before you smoked, so as you can see we are on our way as the first Minor Situational Habit faces the chopping block. You are not fighting your mind, your mind is not your enemy, you are not putting the squeeze on your mind, so your mind will not rebel against this move, your mind knows that you still smoke and that the mother urge is still in place.

You must maintain this behavior as long as it takes to bring your mind to the mental dam construction site, the length of time may differ per person, largely due to how one values their hard earn money, how much money one has at their disposal etc. But sooner or later, hopefully sooner, your mind will arrive at the construction site, do not force the decision, do not make the decision for your mind, I will show you how to deal with a false positive.

The urge underlying the Minor Situational Habit of buying cigarettes is successfully reversed when the 'declination' to throw your hard earned money away outweighs the 'inclination' to buy a pack of cigarettes. Do you see the 'see-saw'?

The behavior of utterly destroying the excess cigarettes peels back the illusion and exposes the naked reality to your mind, the natural conflict between buying cigarettes and throwing your money away, which has always been there, is now literal to your mind.

The behavior constructs the mental dam which is a conflict to be resolved, a problem to be solved, problem solving, conflict resolution is one of your mind's chief functions used to keep a stress free environment.

In order to resolve the stress caused by your insistent behavior of utterly destroying the excess cigarettes your mind goes into problem solving mode, it has only one direction to go based on the construction of the mental dam, it will equate buying cigarettes with throwing your hard earned money away, therefore to stop throwing your hard earned money away it will withdraw or reverse the urge underlying this Minor Situational Habit of buying cigarettes.

But don't get too comfortable, you have been buying cigarettes for years so the urge stretches under that Minor Situational Habit for miles, so the first time you don't feel inclined to buy cigarettes is not cause for celebration just yet, you may experience periodic burps or **false positives** along the way to complete and permanent reversal of that Minor Situational Habit of buying cigarettes.

Let's say after two weeks of this behavior your mind finally forms the equation and responds to the mental dam, you don't feel like buying cigarettes on day 15, now on day 16 you feel an urge to buy a pack of cigarettes, **do not fight this urge**, simply go ahead and buy a pack of cigarettes keeping your ration in mind, so if all you need is one or two cigarettes to complete your daily ration then go ahead and take out that amount.

Yup, you read that right, take out the amount you need to complete your ration even if it is only one cigarette, then utterly destroy the others, the urge will weaken substantially because it is being reversed, think of the urge as a river you are turning, it will take some time to turn, but once it begins to turn it will continue to turn until it is going in the direction the dam is steering it towards, this is no different.

When the urge is completely and permanently reversed the behavior of throwing your hard earned money away will be super-imposed over the act of buying cigarettes, going forward from that point, whenever the mother urge calls buying a pack of cigarettes will not present itself as an option.

Don't be fooled however, the urge is still there and it will present itself eventually, don't fight it when it does, doing so is fighting your mind, and if you do your mind will simply shelf the urge for days, weeks, months, or even years, giving you the impression that you are free of the urge until that day.

Supporting activities:

#1 Daily Ration Maintenance: This is where keeping tabs on your ration comes in, there will be days when you will go over your ration, do not harbor any guilt, remember you are not trying to quit, you are only engaging in behaviors that will construct mental dams nudging your mind in a pre-conceived direction in order to the resolve the conflict it faces.

Let's say your ration is five cigarettes and you smoke six that day, you will subtract one from your next day's ration and only smoke four the next day, that means when you buy a pack of cigarettes you will take out one less than your daily ration. Your goal as it relates to your daily ration is to decrease it comfortably, do not force it, do not start out with a ration you know is impossible to maintain on the first day.

You want to make it challenging but not impossible because your mind will become defensive if you present a challenge to the mother urge, which is to smoke a cigarette.

Let's say your ration is five cigarettes a day and on this particular day you only smoke four, if you maintain that lower amount for two consecutive days then adjust your ration to that lower amount. This is why establishing and monitoring your daily ration is instrumental to your success.

#2 Exercise: Another supporting activity is exercising, whether it's joining a Gym/Spa, or simply power-walking, jogging, cycling, playing tennis, swimming etc. Aerobic exercise is good for the heart and lungs, the more you engage in some form of aerobic exercise the less you will feel like smoking, the mind knows that smoking soon after exercising is like shampooing your white carpet then taking a pound of dirt and garbage and immediately throwing it on your just vacuumed white carpet.

#3 Nutrients: Drink lots of fresh water, eat fresh fruits and vegetables daily. A total body detox is advisable; there are detoxes that are specific to the liver, kidneys etc. Remember you have been and still are ingesting some 7,000+ deadly chemicals, doing all that you can to get them out of your body is a plus.

#4 Language: The proper use of language during the construction of the mental dams is very crucial. You are not smoking a cigarette, you are smoking an arsenic laced cancer stick, a cancer stick dipped in formaldehyde, a cancer stick containing ammonia and carbon monoxide.

Tell yourself the truth as you engage in the behavior, remind your mind of the actual reality it has created a comfort zone around. So go ahead light up that cancer stick containing over 7,000+ deadly poisonous toxins, after all your car's tailpipe is too big and uncomfortable for your mouth.

#5 Smoke free zones: You now know about 2nd and 3rd hand smoke, you know that when you smoke around others, especially those that do not themselves smoke cancer sticks, that the smoke coming off the tip is unfiltered and thus the full 7,000+ chemical poisons are being ingested by those around you. You know that when you pick up your daughter and hold her close to you that the smoke in your hair and clothes containing traces of those 7,000+ chemical poisons are going into her little, fragile, still forming lungs and brain.

You did not begin this habit to kill others, but inadvertently the facts are the facts, so now that you know, establish smoke-free zones, limit where you will and won't smoke, keep the health of your children, friends, co-workers, and family in mind.

By establishing smoke-free zones this will also decrease when the mind will present the urge to you, remember, one of your mind's duties is to protect you from stress, so just as it does not present you with the urge to smoke while asleep, or in the hospital, or sitting in the pews at a church, it won't present the urge when you are in one of your defined smoke-free zones.

If you have children at home, or if your wife or husband or other family members do not smoke and they live with you, then zone your home smoke-free. If you live alone but you get the children every other weekend, then every other weekend when your children are with you zone your home smoke-free, you may even go so far as to zone the week-end smoke-free, keeping 3rd hand smoke in mind.

Mental Dam #2

Now that you no longer feel the urge to engage the first Minor Situational Habit of buying cigarettes, the second Minor Situational Habit of 'bumming' will move forward as the means by which the mother urge is maintained.

By the time you get to this step your daily ration should have decreased noticeably. You are exercising more, walking, running, biking, swimming, aerobics, these are all great exercises to flush the lungs and create a sense of well-being.

Since the Major Situational Habit, the act of smoking a cigarette, is still in place you will now find yourself acquiring the cigarette by the second Minor Situational Habit of 'Bumming'.

This was formerly a low-key act but with the reversal of the urge to buy cigarettes, which was the first option, this Minor Situational Habit now moves up as the first option. It will also increase in frequency according to your daily ration. This Minor Situational Habit comes with its own parameters, depending on the type of person you are you may not be comfortable just 'bumming' a cigarette from just anyone. During this phase I personally bummed only from the few friends, and co-workers who smoked cigarettes.

Some people are very comfortable bumming from just about anyone, if you fall in this category don't worry, I got you, this mental dam I'm about to introduce to you works no matter if you bum from a selective few or if you bum from anyone around you.

Objective: To construct a mental dam using the attitudes of others towards having their hard earned money thrown away. By using this technique, we will effectively diminish the pool of persons that will cater to your bumming, it's one thing to throw your hard earned money away, it's quite another to throw someone else's hard earned money away.

Method: Bum a cigarette from someone who is stationary and more likely smoking, this may typically be in a defined smoking area while on break, or it may be at a social event. The key is you want the person you are bumming from to see what you do with the cigarette you just bummed from them, so bumming from someone who will not witness what you do with their hard earned money will not garner the full impact.

Now that you have bummed the cigarette go ahead and light up, take 2 or three puffs then right in front of the person you just bummed from, drop the remainder of the cigarette and step on it, if you are indoors and only have access to an ashtray then squash the remainder of the cigarette practically smashing it to bits, you get the picture, if there is an empty beer bottle or such then you may drop the cigarette in, the idea is to only take a few puffs then literally discard the remainder right in front of the person you just bummed from.

Most people will not tolerate it, especially with the rising cost of cigarettes, some people may become downright agitated with you, that's to be expected, use this to your advantage, these are people who will soon stop allowing you to bum from them.

Some people may want to charge you to bum from them once they witness what you actually do with their hard earned money, follow the same process of taking only a few puffs then discarding the remainder, your mind is already reversing the urge to buy cigarettes, you no longer buy packs of cigarettes, so if you do buy a loosie (one cigarette) don't panic, go ahead and throw your hard earned money away after 2 or 3 puffs.

If during this 'bumming' phase you feel an urge to buy a pack or some 'loosies' don't fight the urge, if you buy a pack take out the one cigarette you need and utterly destroy the remainder, that's right, do not take out your ration from the pack, if you are down to about 3 or 4 cigarettes a day, at this stage of 'bumming' should the urge to buy a pack present itself go ahead and do so, but only take out the one cigarette you need right then and there and utterly destroy the remainder. By doing this you further reinforce the mental dam and strengthen your mind's reversal of that urge, it won't be long before the thought of buying a pack of cigarettes never occur to you again.

Supporting Activity: Your ongoing supporting activity of exercising, drinking lots of fresh water, eating fruits and vegetables should in and of themselves become habitual to you by now, you are showing love to yourself in a very real way. You may not have thought about it this way but cigarette smoking has altered your lifestyle from a healthy one to an unhealthy one, you are re-constructing a healthy lifestyle for yourself.

The specific supporting activity of 'language' is highly beneficial to you during this step. Remember the objective is to encourage those you bum from to rightfully cut you off. When you bum a cigarette now don't just ask for a cigarette, instead ask for a 'cancer stick', or you may say something like 'do you have another arsenic laced cigarette to spare?', what you are doing is turning the person you are bumming from off, it won't be long before they cut you off.

When you use this degree of truthful language you are also presenting the truth to your mind which is currently trapped in an illusion, you are reminding your mind of the actual reality. So instead of telling yourself you're going to have a cigarette, tell yourself you are going to suck some carbon monoxide and ammonia into your lungs, then go ahead and light up.

Results

This technique also sets up a conflict that the mind is obligated to resolve. Depending on your character, you may not be comfortable bumming from anyone, after all 'a bum is a bum is a bum', combine this with the guilt you will produce when you actually throw someone else's hard earned money away. You have your integrity and your character to protect, you will not want to be branded a bum, a cheapskate, disrespectful etc.

Fairly soon the act of 'bumming' will become a burden to you and the people you bum from. You know very well that no one likes to support another person's bad habits. You will see the subtle and not so subtle signs of irritability from those who really don't want you to bum from them, use this to your advantage, so as not to damage relationships discontinue bumming from those persons, your mind will be leading the way on this because this is the direction the mental dam is steering it towards.

To resolve the conflict caused by the construction of this mental dam, your mind will lessen and eventually reverse the urge to bum a cigarette. Your pool may be one or two people at this time, continue to drive that wedge, even though they may know what you are doing, the fact is you're still literally throwing their hard earned money away.

When your daily ration is one or two cigarettes it is time to construct the final mental dam. The success of the final step relies heavily on your successful construction of the first two mental dams.

<u>Clear The Smoke</u>

Before we go into the final step and construct the final mental dam, let's recap the expected results of the first two steps, remember, this is not a sprint, most, if not all of you have been smoking since you were teenagers, you may now be twenty-something, thirty-something, or even seventy-something.

This is not an overnight process, but it will be a permanent process with no negative side effects, if the steps are adhered to as presented in this book, no short-cuts, you don't have to be a student or professional in the Behavioral Sciences, you weren't one when you started and you don't need a degree to successfully reverse the bad habit your mind has built a comfort zone around.

The Tobacco Industrial Complex and its after-market Big Pharma and the Medical Industrial Complex will try to convince you that you cannot get rid of this habit without them, they will throw terms like 'endorphins, dopamine' etc at you in order to convince you that the problem is more physiological than psychological, just remember, no matter how many cigarettes you smoke during the day you still go to sleep at night for between 4-8 hours, and you do not jump up out of your sleep every hour to feed an endorphin rush.

The first **Minor Situational Habit**, which is the act of buying cigarettes, is successfully 'dammed' when the 'declination' to throw your hard earned money away outweighs your 'inclination' to buy a pack of cigarettes. The consistent behavior of extracting your daily ration and utterly destroying the remainder has constructed the first mental dam.

This first mental dam revealed the literal conflict between buying cigarettes and throwing your hard earned money away. To resolve this conflict your mind naturally and without force has formed the association that in order to **stop throwing your hard earned money away, you must stop buying cigarettes.** Your mind cannot force you to buy or not buy cigarettes, it only controls the urge which is like the current under the wave, so your mind will begin to reverse the urge to buy cigarettes which will naturally strengthen the 'declination' end and weaken the 'inclination' end of the see-saw.

This first mental dam construction will take as long as you are comfortable with literally throwing your hard earned money away. As stated before this is not for those who have money to burn, but most of us work very hard for our money.

Due to not fighting the urge, but consistently destroying the excess cancer sticks, your mind has unequivocally concluded that if ever you buy a pack of cigarettes you will literally throw your money away.

By the time you have moved into the construction of the second dam your ration should have decreased, you are exercising more, eating fresh fruits (which helps the body eliminate toxins), drinking lots of fresh water (I recommend alkaline water), you have established smoke-free zones keeping 2nd and 3rd hand smoke in mind, and you are telling your mind the truth about what you are really doing, your language is harsh, you aren't just going to have a smoke, you are going to suck on a cancer stick laced with arsenic, ammonia and formaldehyde just to name a few of the 7,000+ chemical poisons found in cigarettes.

The second **Minor Situational Habit,** which is the act of bumming, is now the chief means by which the mother urge is engaged. You arrived at this point because you no longer buy cigarettes, which means you are naturally smoking less, and the mother urge, which is the urge to incline to smoke, is weakening.

You successfully constructed this 2nd mental dam with the deliberate and consistent behavior of taking a few puffs of the cancer stick you just bummed and destroying the remainder, right in front of the person you bummed it from.

This behavior naturally decreased the pool of persons you feel comfortable bumming from, by continuing the behavior you advertently eliminate or justifiably irritate the few remaining persons from that pool.

Your use of 'mind-awakening language' is especially useful here as you bum cancer sticks laced with arsenic, your mind is unraveling itself from the illusion it is trapped in, your daily ration is drastically reduced, you are exercising, eating lots of fresh fruits and vegetables, drinking fresh water daily, in effect you are daily flushing the harmful 7,000+ chemical toxins from your systems.

Your declination to smoke is beginning to outweigh your inclination to smoke, this is happening naturally, no force, your mental dams are having the desired effects of turning the mother urge, which can be likened to a mighty river, the see-saw teeters.

Mental Dam #3

In the beginning this was the Major Situational Habit, the mother habit, the act of smoking cigarettes, undergirded by the mother urge, the urge to incline you to smoke cigarettes. Remember, the mind is not hooked on the act of smoking, it is hooked on the urge to smoke, it is the current that moves the waves, not the waves themselves.

Now that your mind has reversed the urge on the two supporting Minor Situational Habits, the Major Situational Habit has been reduced to a Minor Situational Habit, it has been substantially weakened, at this point you will drive the final nail in, you will zap this habit like the bug it is, you will once and for all take your mind back from being the footstool to an urge to kill yourself and those around you, you will no longer commit suicide by cigarette.

Objective: To cause your mind to permanently reverse the urge to incline you to smoke cigarettes. Like a river that has been dammed into making a U-turn, the urge to incline to smoke cigarettes is on its way back out of your mind, not on a high shelf waiting for that day, but permanently removed from every crack and crevice of your mind.

The Method: This is known as the 'do as you say' method, let me qualify this will work for you because you are a person of self-esteem, integrity, and great character, your word is your bond, you will not allow yourself to be viewed as a hypocrite, a liar, someone who says one thing but does the opposite, if this is not who you are then this method may not work for you.

One of the main duties of your mind is to protect your 'ego' from shame and negative stress. When faced with a conflict your mind will always seek to resolve the conflict in favor of preserving your pride, your ego-self, the conscious part of you that you think people see when they look at you. This is what we will activate fully as we construct this final mental dam.

You are at a party, bar, nightclub, family reunion, office party, or any group setting, people are drinking and smoking, you know how inclined you are to smoke when you drink, smoke when others are smoking, smoke when you are chatting, smoke when you are eating, the social group setting is the perfect mini-situation where the mother urge is at an inclination buffet.

Before you started applying the steps in this book you would easily smoke about double your daily amount at one of these settings, just about every conceivable mini-situations presents itself at these types of settings, that's why I labeled it '**an inclination buffet**'.

At these settings you smoke with every beer or drink, you smoke after eating chicken wings, you smoke because the person that just joined you lights up, even though you just got thru smoking, you smoke when you go to the rest room, you smoke when you go outside, you smoke when you come back in, you smoke, you smoke, you smoke.

Just think, if your mind curbs the urge to smoke in this environment, you will be well on your way to never smoking cigarettes again.

The technique is very simple, when you first arrive at the scene target a few strangers and friends, engage them in conversation about the hazards of smoking cigarettes, make a really big deal about it, you must be very convincing, your position is, you no longer smoke cigarettes and will not be caught dead sucking on those disgusting cancer sticks.

Talk about the hazards of 2nd and 3rd hand smoke, people must be convinced that you are dead set against smoking, and you are, you are not lying, you are taking a position publicly that your mind will have to support in order to preserve your self-dignity, in order to protect your ego-self from shame. It is a position you are now prepared to claim.

Continue this line of conversation whenever the opportunity arises with as many strangers and friends as possible. The reason why you must choose strangers is because you never know where they may see you next, even though they may not recognize you if they saw you again, your mind will not take that chance.

Your behavior constructs the final dam in which your mind must choose between the urge to incline to smoke and your public image, how you are perceived, protecting your ego-self from shame. The conflict will look like this to your mind:

- You can sneak off to the bathroom and light one up in the privacy of the stall, but one of those people that witnessed the statement 'I will not be caught dead smoking one of those cancer sticks' may come into the bathroom just as you are coming out of the stall, they may smell the smoke on your breath. You will be seen as a hypocrite and a liar.

- Or the mind will suspend the urge to smoke in that environment, just as it does when you are asleep, or in an environment where it will cause you great stress to engage the urge to incline to smoke. So you will go thru the densest environment where multiple mini-situations exist, you will drink and don't feel like smoking, you will eat and don't feel like smoking, you will engage in chatting, you will see other people smoke and you will not feel like smoking. Not because you are being defiant as you struggle against your mind, but because you and your mind are working together and your mind is responding to this mental dam by severely curbing the urge to incline you to smoke. In fact, you may not feel like staying in a smoke-filled environment and be subject to 2nd hand smoke.

Even after you have left the party, continue this line of conversation wherever you frequent, wherever you usually smoked, the barbershop, beauty salon, the job, the mall etc. You will not feel the urge to smoke even at home, what if someone drops by and smells the smoke, you will not smoke in your car, what if someone sees you or smells the smoke. When you travel long distance, follow the same technique, whether you travel to another country on vacation, engage the bellhop, the hotel desk clerk, the cab driver, your mind will do the rest.

Your behavior has constructed the mental dam that steers your mind in the only possible direction, to completely reverse the urge to incline you to smoke cigarettes. You will be back on the otherside where the 'inclination' is dangling in the air and your 'declination' is firmly grounded, your declination continues to get heavier with each passing mini-situation where the urge to incline is overpowered by the urge to decline.

You used to have a cigarette right after you eat, you used to light up just before going to bed, or with your morning coffee, now the urge to incline is a faint echo getting fainter and fainter until the last of the mother urge trickles out of your mind.

You made it, your mind is now permanently free of the urge to incline to smoke cancer sticks, you have crossed back over to where you were before you ever smoked, the same feelings of disgust at the thought of smoking is still there, you look at cigarette smoking with disdain, you feel sorry for those who are trapped.

The big difference is that you have the experience of what it means to be trapped, but now that you are no longer in your peer pressure years, there is nothing heavy enough to outweigh your declination, because this declination, unlike the original, comes with experience, so it weighs a couple of tons, it will not be moved, as a matter of fact your declination stands alone, there is no inclination to oppose it, there is no longer a see-saw because sucking on those disgusting cancer sticks laced with over 7,000+ deadly chemical toxins like:

- o **carbon monoxide** (car exhaust)
- o **tar** (makes roads)
- o **arsenic** (rat poison)
- o **ammonia** (cleaning products)

- o **hydrogen cyanide** (gas chamber poison)
- o **cyanide**
- o **acetone** (nail polish remover)
- o **butane** (lighter fluid)
- o **DDT** (insecticide)
- o **formaldehyde** (embalm fluid)
- o **sulfuric acid** (car battery)
- o **lead**

Just to name a few, is no longer an option. You safely reversed the habit without the use of drugs and the many side effects, you did it with your mind not against it, hence it is permanent. **You can say you made up your mind.**

After The Smoke Clears

Quitting is not a permanent fix, in fact you quit every night you go to bed. When you quit you merely suspend the habit, the see-saw does not reverse, it remains with your declination dangling in the air, and your inclination grounded. You may suspend or freeze this picture for a very long time, weeks, months, even years, but all it takes is the right trigger, maybe the loss of a loved one, a divorce, loss of a job, some intense pressure or maybe no pressure.

Maybe the mood was just right, a few drinks, everyone else smoking, maybe you met someone you really want to be with and they smoke, it can be anything at anytime that causes the picture to unfreeze and you will pick up exactly where you left off.

When you reverse the habit, which is what you have done using this book, you reverse the see-saw in your mind, the urge to decline to smoke outweighs your urge to incline to smoke. You cross back over to the side where cigarette smoke was repulsive to you, you would have never smoked were it not for the external inducements like peer pressure, the need to fit in, that sat on the side of the urge to incline over and over again until the habit of inclining was formed.

But now you have the experience, you are no longer naïve to the reality of smoking cigarettes, you are fully aware of the real danger it poses not only to yourself but to everyone around you thru 2nd and 3rd hand smoke. You have developed a healthier lifestyle, you enjoy breathing without coughing, fresh air tastes really good to you.

The Major Situational Habit, which is the urge to incline to smoke, has been effectively reduced to a very weak Minor Situational Habit due to the construction of mental dams then permanently reversed out of your mind.

Welcome to the remainder of your smoke-free life, because of using the methods in this book you did not have to contend with any unwanted side effects such as abnormal weight gain, sleepless nights, irritability, nausea or other effects produced when your mind is forced to do something it has not resolved to do.

Instead you have experienced a guilt free journey back to your beginning and have successfully crossed back over. **You made it, you and your mind together, partners, the way it is intended to be**. Congratulations

DAM

DAM THAT HABIT

HABIT

www.ingramcontent.com/pod-product-compliance
Lightning Source LLC
Chambersburg PA
CBHW050540270326
41926CB00015B/3325